Hi, My Name Is Kim.....

a story of breast cancer and media survival

By Kim Friedrich

© 2008 Kim Friedrich

Hi, My Name Is Kim…
A Story Of Breast Cancer And Media
Survival
Copyright © 2008 by Kim Friedrich

Summary: The true story of all the thoughts and feelings, both physical and emotional, that one woman went through during the diagnosis and chemo process with regards to breast cancer.
ISBN 978-0-6152-1175-6
Non-Fiction

CHAPTERS

Ch. 1

INTRODUCTION

"Hi, my name is Kim, I'm 36 years old, and hope to be a future breast cancer survivor from Long Island."

This is how the world learned of my existence. I've always dreamed of becoming a senator and helping people, but apparently that's a game only the rich get to play, and when they get there they seem to forget they did it to help people. I'd like to have been known for sponsoring legislation to save Social Security, to promote solar power, to greatly decrease the number of uninsured in our country, but that's not likely to happen.

As I sit putting fingers to keyboard (who uses pen and paper anymore), it is estimated that 47 million people in this country are without medical insurance. When my story began, I was one of them, as were my husband and children. We were one part of the unlucky masses that got caught up in corporate downsizing. My husband went for a year and a half without finding a real job. Oh he had temp jobs at call centers but the pay is incredibly low and there are no benefits. He went on a million interviews, but nothing panned out. I was the office manager at Temple Beth Chai in Hauppauge, NY. My parents have belonged to that Temple since I was 2 years old and I loved working there but I had to find a full time job that paid more and provided benefits. It took me about 7 months but I found a position. Somebody explain to me again about how great this economy is, because somehow it's passing me by.

Anyway, my reason for writing this is two-fold:

#1 to help people.

One thing I found in going through this process of discovery was that I felt as though no one was answering my questions. Whenever and whatever I asked the answer was always the same "well everyone is different". Guess what doc's… that doesn't help.

#2 to show you that you're not alone.

Even if you don't learn anything about the chemotherapy process, maybe there will be a moment where you realize that you or someone very close to you may be feeling something I felt. You are not alone in your feelings. Feelings are as important as facts, when it comes to cancer.

If I reach one person, and help her to push on with her treatment, this will all have been worth it.

Ch. 2

BEFORE CANCER

My story begins back in October 2005. That was when my husband, Matt, lost his job. He was making a decent, but not great salary when you take into account commuting costs to Manhattan. But he had been with his company for 4 years; everything seemed to be going well, and with the economy the way it was he was afraid to be found looking for another job.

We had bought a house the year before. When we were looking, we had to take many factors into account. There was his job in New York City, my job on Long Island (moderate paying but steady), the fact that we had one child with special needs and another on the way, and that my mother was our primary day care provider. If we moved to New Jersey or Pennsylvania, I would have to find another job, we would have to pay for daycare, and we would have no friends and family in close driving distance if there were problems. When taking all that into account, we decided to buy the cheapest fixer-upper on Long Island we could find. A fixer upper on Long Island costs $250,000.

Now we have a house, a mortgage that costs about $1,780 / month, and Matt's commuting cost is about $300/month and 4 ½ hours each day. That's everyday folks. He gets up before dawn and gets back after dark just to keep us in a house.

Then he loses his job. The Information Technology Department cut back from three employees to two, and since he was neither the supervisor, nor the lowest paid, he got the axe. Along with his job went our health insurance. Of course we could not afford COBRA. I don't even know who can afford this once they lose their job. When you lose your job, you lose your income. How you are supposed to pay $1,000ish a month for health insurance is beyond me.

We looked into NYS child health plus to at least cover the kids, but every time Matt would get some crummy part time or temp job for extra money, we would be over the limit. In fact we were over the limit for food stamps too. Let's do the math. I was making $12/hour, 30 hours a week. That's $1,440 / month. My husband would get temp jobs often also paying $12/hour 40 hours a week. That's $1,920 a month for a total of $3,360/month. Of course that's before taxes, but that's what the limit goes by. The limit in NY for a family of 4 to receive food stamps was $2,097/month. So on $3,360, which was more like $2,300 after taxes, with $1,780 going for the house alone, the highest electricity rates in the country, oil skyrocketing and we have an oil burner, and all the other expenses of just living... we can't get food stamps or free health insurance for the kids, let alone us.

Now we are approaching the end of February 2007. Land taxes have gone up dramatically so now our mortgage costs $2,200/month. Nobody is helping us besides various family members throwing us what money they can. A job is nowhere in sight for my husband. Credit card bills are piling up into the tens of thousands (its amazing how having to charge food, heating oil and gas adds up). And then one morning I wake up, and find the problem to trump all other problems.

Ch. 3

THAT FATEFUL MORNING

I woke up and my chest hurt. Not a lot, but like I bruised my ribs in my sleep or something. I reached over to my left side to touch my rib… and I felt it. A lump. Now I'm not a genius, but I know that's not supposed to be there.

It felt huge, as if it was taking up most of the left side of my left breast. I went into the bathroom and looked at myself in the mirror. I started playing with my breast; after all maybe it wasn't really a lump. Maybe it was something pliable. Maybe something just got stuck in there for a second. But no, it was a lump.

I can't explain why, but I knew it was cancer. Even though nobody in my family has cancer except some extremely distant aunt twice removed or something, I knew it was cancer. As this realization hit me, I just locked myself in the bathroom and cried.

Not long after that my husband, Matt, woke up. He was getting our older girl ready for school because he didn't have any interviews that day. I, on the other hand, had to get ready for work. I couldn't tell him what was wrong. Not yet. It was too soon. But I didn't know what to do or, for that matter, where to go.

When I got to work that day, I called Planned Parenthood and made an appointment. I just didn't know where else to turn. I didn't even think about clinics or going to the emergency room. This wasn't an emergency right? I got an appointment for 4 days later. Four days of hell… before the rest of the hell. But there was nothing I could do but wait at this point. I hardly did anything at work that day, I just couldn't focus. I wouldn't really say I was thinking about what to tell Matt either. It was as though I stopped thinking. Then I looked up and it was 3pm and time to go home.

I walked in the door and he was downstairs playing solitaire on his computer. As I walked down to the basement I asked how his day was. It was obviously bad because he started yelling at me. "One call back, one freaking call back and that was to tell me no thanks", or something along those lines. I looked at him with tears in my eyes and he assured me that someone would call; he'd have a job soon. It was like one of those misunderstandings out of a movie and I almost laughed at that thought. Instead I told him why I was crying.

Matt just looked at me asking if I'm sure, and I let him touch the lump. Its funny how a man who has touched my breasts who knows how many times over the almost 12 years we were married at that point, could be so afraid to touch them at that moment. He felt it, and asked if I was sure it was a lump. I told him I've never felt it before, that it's something new in my breast. Then I told him about my appointment with Planned Parenthood and we agreed not to talk about it again until after I saw them. After all, 4 days wouldn't change anything. The thing is, that's what it would seem like every step of this process would be. Just 4 more days, just another week, just 6 more treatments. The word "just" became the most hated and then months later the most loved word in my house.

As each day started, I'd say to myself "just 3 more days, just 2 more days" and as they ended "just 2 ½ more days, just 1

½ more days". Each day itself would drag on. Just 3 more hours until lunch. Just 2 more hours until I get to go home… and count just how many hours it is until I put the kids to bed. By the time Friday arrived, I was manic. Just how long until my appointment? 90 minutes. Ok I can make it just 90 minutes more. Of course I couldn't wait and arrived 30 minutes early. Now I have to sit and wait in their waiting room. I'm just glad it has a TV on; at least I can watch "The View".

By the time they call my name, I was sitting in tears again. I wasn't even sure why I was crying, but I couldn't stop. I was brought into a room and got my act together, told them that I felt a lump and didn't know what to do. Three nurses and a doctor felt my breast and all agreed; yes it was a lump of some kind. Couldn't tell what kind, of course, but they did their part. I'm not nuts, there definitely is something there.

Here is where Planned Parenthood went into overdrive. I can never thank them enough, because they could see I was lost, had no health insurance, and didn't know what to do. They contacted the Women's Health Partnership of Suffolk County, which I had never heard of before. Hopefully you all have a Women's Health Partnership (WHP) in your state. They would pay for all my medical needs through diagnosis, and then they would help me get on a Medicaid program to pay for the rest. I was stunned. I still am, because, while my bills were piling up with no end in sight and both my husband and I were still looking for jobs, at least this would be covered. It was a Godsend.

Planned Parenthood gave me a prescription for a sonogram and while I was there the WHP made an appointment for me to see a surgeon. Unfortunately she couldn't see me for a week but I could go that day for the sonogram. I had never had a breast sonogram before; I didn't even realize that you did them on breasts. I knew about mammograms of course, but not sonograms. But that's what they wanted... so that's what I got. I went to a lab, they called WHP to confirm payment (because it's all about money of course), and in I went. After it was done I had to wait for a doctor to look at the results. This was the first time I felt like I would have something concrete about my health. Of course I was hoping he would come out and say that it was just a hard cyst, but no chance. The doctor told me on a scale of 0-4, with 4 being the most suspicious, he would put it at about a 3.5.

At this point all I could do was wait to see the surgeon. Once again, it was just 6 more days, then just 4 more nights.... I hated just. The second I met her, I hated her office. I hated that I had to go to a different window from everyone else because of being on a "special program", but at least I was getting to see a doctor, right? The woman seemed very nice, and I'm sure competent, but I could have ripped her head off anyway. Matt and I were with her for about 5 minutes. She looked at the sonogram and felt my breast. Then she told me that she wanted me to do a mammogram and we'd schedule a date for surgery. SURGERY?? Wait, I'm here 5 minutes. Don't you want to talk to me some more? Ask me more questions? Do more tests? A biopsy? SOMETHING?

What she told me was that she could almost guarantee that this was cancer, and she wanted to do a lumpectomy to determine if it was malignant and remove the growth all at the same time. Well ok, that makes sense, I told myself.

But what then if it is malignant? Well then she recommends removing the entire breast, and because it looks like it's in the milk ducts already, I may want to remove my right one as a precaution. At this point my head was spinning. I took the prescription for the mammogram and left. I didn't even hear the rest of what she said, Matt had to tell me. She wanted me to call immediately after having the mammogram to schedule the surgery.

This is a very important lesson by the way. I highly recommend always bringing someone with you to every appointment with every doctor, or at the very least bring a notebook. Write everything down and ask the doctor if you missed anything. When you are dealing with life or death issues, and the word CANCER strikes a dread in people so strong it can cause hysterical deafness, you need a way to hear everything that is being said.

So here I go, once again to the lab. This time, when I arrived, they actually asked me to make an appointment. No problem, I was getting used to that. So three days later I have my first mammogram.

Ch. 4

DAYS PASS BY

So, mammogram done, same result. 3.5.

At this point, I give the surgeon a call. She can't see me for at least 6 weeks for surgery. 6 weeks?? I'm sitting here dying of cancer (probably) and I have to wait? Yep, that's what I'm told. Well I make the appointment and fume.

On Monday I have a job interview. It is an industry in which I have an extensive background. I just knew I could nail it. Problem is, I could be sitting there with cancer. If they knew that, they would never hire me. I don't know if legally they could turn me down, but they would anyway. I'd all of a sudden be unqualified.

Well, the interview went swimmingly, I knew the job was mine. The people seemed very nice, funny, and it would be a comfortable fit for me. Not a tremendous amount more per hour to start, but it would be full time instead of 30 hours a week and after 3 months I'd have health insurance. I had to keep my fingers crossed that everything would go well with the biopsy. It was just killing me to wait 6 weeks.

I called back the Women's Health Partnership and asked if I could see another doctor. They made a bunch of calls and found a plastic surgeon who would see me that day. My Mom jumped into her car and drove me to his office (she has been my rock through all this). I brought my mammogram and sonogram films to show him, he felt my breast, and agreed with me, I shouldn't wait. However, he also agreed with the first surgeon. He said we must do a lumpectomy, or at least partial lumpectomy, and use that for the biopsy. For future reference, insist on a core biopsy first... I'll explain why soon.

He worked out of an ambulatory surgical center and Matt and I went down there the very next day. It didn't seem to take very long, just a few hours. I was booked for a follow up appointment for Thursday, although the biopsy results might not be back yet. When I got to his office (Mom drove me again), he told me that while he did not have the results of the biopsy, he knows what cancer looks like. This is definitely cancer. At this point, we needed to schedule a mastectomy, because that's standard procedure in a case as advanced as mine. He estimated it was about 4cm in diameter and in the milk ducts, although he saw no signs of it in my lymph nodes.

Ch. 5

THE PEOPLE YOU LOVE

While all this is going on, its tough to keep things away from people you've known your whole life. Truth is, maybe you shouldn't keep things from them. There is a reason they've been in your life that long, because they're good people who want to be there for you in good times and bad.

I didn't want people from my Temple to know. It doesn't matter that I've known many of them since before I could walk. I just couldn't face them. I couldn't face the "oh I'm so sorry" and "if there is anything I can do". But a Temple isn't just a group of people, it's a family all of whom have their own stories and problems and things they have overcome. One of the most special members to me was Penny. Penny is a breast cancer survivor. In fact she had breast cancer almost identical to mine. But she isn't the kind of woman who just did what doctors said. She researched. She wanted the best of the best working on her... doesn't everyone? She kept pushing and pushing for me to see her surgeon. Not only did he save her life and her breasts, he actually saved her fertility. Well I didn't want more kids, but I thought how remarkable that was. I had always heard that once you had chemo that was it, no more kids. If this doctor was good enough for her, he was good enough for me. I called him up, and miracle of miracles, he had a cancellation. I was able to see him a few days after I had my biopsy.

During this time, I was offered the job for which I interviewed. I accepted it, but told them I couldn't start for 2 ½ weeks to give time for my Temple to find a replacement. I also needed to buy time to find out if I had cancer. Well now I knew, I had it. So here I am, a new hire who hasn't started yet, going in and telling my would-be bosses that I have just been diagnosed with breast cancer. I'm crying in the manager's office. I tell her and the assistant manager that it's up to them if they still want to give me the job. I understand if they don't, because there is no way this cannot affect my job, but that given time off for treatment I will be an excellent employee. At this point as I write this, I've been an employee of Suffolk Federal Credit Union for 6 months. They have been wonderful, accommodating, caring, everything you think employers can't be nowadays.

Also, the Women's Health Partnership got me onto Medicaid. Apparently there is a program in New York that allows you to have medical costs paid if you make less then three times the poverty level and are already diagnosed with breast cancer. Now that is a big thing, you must already be diagnosed. How many women don't go to doctors because they don't have health insurance? How many forgo mammograms that might find lumps when they're too small to feel, just because they can't afford them? For that matter, how many of these women know this program exists? I didn't. I'm grateful it does, but only covering medical costs once you have a diagnosis of breast cancer may mean more invasive, costly treatment for many women. If diagnostic tests were covered by Medicaid, breast cancer would be caught in much earlier stages... but that might be too close to socialized medicine and that would be bad, right?

Now the hard part to write about, the daydreams and nightmares. I've always been a person who dreams, but my dreams aren't very detailed, more like a short scene from a

TV show. They would last 1 minute at the most, at least that's all I can remember. Doesn't matter if it's a daydream or night dream. Good dreams and bad, all are short.

One day near the end of my tenure at Temple Beth Chai, as I'm driving home, I start to daydream while driving. I see myself sick in bed, almost unrecognizable. I'm hairless, white as snow, thin to the point of seeing my bones sticking out of me, everything I'm not. My husband is sitting next to me crying. I tell him to take care of the kids and the scene goes dark. Naturally I start crying. For the next 15 minutes or so on the way home, I cry realizing that I just told my husband goodbye. That at least for that brief moment, the realization sunk in that I could die.

This wasn't a one time occurrence. For the next 3 months or so, every once in a while for no reason, I'd have a goodbye scene play out. Sometimes a bit longer then others, those usually happened at night. But I said goodbye to my parents, my best friends Ivy and Paulette, Matt countless times, the kids…. pretty much everyone I've ever met. I'd dream these scenes over and over like they were rehearsals. As if someday I'd get them perfected so I could eventually say it for real.

The more I had them, the more I feared having them. The more I feared having them, the more I seemed to have them. It was a vicious cycle. There were times when it seemed as though I were playing out one of these scenes everyday. The worst part was that the longer this went on and the more perfected my goodbyes to each one became, the less I saw myself in the dream. Instead of it being as though I were watching a scene on TV, I started seeing the scene happening through my eyes. So I could see Matt, Mom, et al, looking down at my obviously sickly face with tears in their eyes as I'm talking to them. I wanted these dreams to stop and I wanted them to stop now. I just hoped at some point to figure out a way.

Ch. 6

A NEW DOCTOR, A NEW BEGINNING

So there we are, Mom driving me 3 hours (or what became 3 hours because of torrential rain) to go see Penny's doctor. It was worth the wait.

Initially I didn't want to go to him. He was too far away; I'd be too far away from everyone if he rushed me into surgery, etc. Well ya know what; my advice is to go with the best. Don't shortchange yourself. The guy I saw is the head of the breast cancer department at a major medical center in New York. He works in a team philosophy, many different specialists all in different facets of breast cancer working together. He is strictly a breast cancer surgeon. If anyone could make sure the cancer was taken out of a breast without removing too much excess tissue, this was the guy.

I get in there 9 days after the partial lumpectomy. My breast is aching, and the ache is getting worse everyday, but I figure it's just because I had surgery 9 days before. I had called the plastic surgeon about it, but he said not to be concerned and to have the breast surgeon look at it, but it is probably just my skin trying to heal. Anyway, I get in and the office is the most beautiful doctor's office I've ever seen. I know, a pretty office doesn't make for a good doctor, but it was just soooo nice. After a bit we meet the doctor and his assistant and he looks at my breast and is very concerned. He asks for a razor to cut open the stitching and squeezes my breast. Well, out from the freshly sliced cut, pours puss. It doesn't just pour, it actually spurts. It's like something from a bad horror movie. Buckets. They're bringing in towels to soak it up off the floor. My Mom, who is in the room with me, is staring stunned. She can't get over how much is spouting out of me. I tell him what my previous surgeon said. This doctor tells me that in another couple of days I would have been in the emergency room with 105 degree fever. Considering that in a matter of minutes the doctor's floor is so covered with liquid it takes several towels (not paper towels, big full towels) to clean it up, I find it hard not to agree with him. So the doc gives me a shot of antibiotic and cleans it with some iodine, and we go on to discuss my case. He looks at my film, looks in the fresh cut to get a glimpse, and has me dress to meet him in his office.

No decisions will be made until after he can talk to his team, but he thinks he can save my breast. He tells me that, statistically, there is no difference in the mortality rate between a lumpectomy and a mastectomy. The only reason to do a mastectomy is cosmetic. If you have to remove so much tissue from one breast that it becomes noticeably smaller that the other breast you are better off in doing a mastectomy followed by reconstructive surgery. The one hiccup is the fact that I had a partial lumpectomy instead of a core biopsy. In a core biopsy, a tube is inserted through a very small incision, and it takes out a portion of the lump down to its core. This way many layers of the lump can be examined because not every lump is cancerous through and though. Just part may be. However, by making a 2 ½ inch incision in my breast, the plastic surgeon cut may have disturbed the blood supply to the lump. He may have blown my shot at doing chemo first, before any further surgery. The idea of doing chemo before surgery is a new concept. The theory behind it is that it can reduce the lump to a manageable size, thereby saving the breast. He would meet with his team next Tuesday to discuss the matter with them.

Ultimately, whatever was decided he assured me that he would save my life. I can't say if it's because he was a specialist, or just supremely confident, but immediately I felt better. This was the doctor for me. Thanks again Penny.

Well Tuesday rolls around, no call. I try not to panic, but I'm afraid my case is forgotten about because I have no insurance. No worries though, his assistant calls on Wednesday afternoon. The team decided ironically, because I had the raging infection, there is so much blood pumping through my breast that I'm still a good candidate. Yeah, luck is on my side for a change. We discuss options, and traveling to the city for every treatment just isn't workable. So he gives me the name of a few oncologist / hematologists closer to home, and I check with Penny and find that one of them is the one she went to. Well that's the doctor for me!

Ch. 7

A PORT, YOUR VEIN'S BEST FRIEND

So it's the middle of May 2007 and I'm going to begin treatment soon. My doctor wants me to have a port surgically implanted. A port is a device through which the medication can be administered without having to go into veins. I wasn't exactly crazy about the idea of having surgery, but since I had heard that chemo can really do damage to people's veins, this port thing sounded like a good idea.

I have to tell you, there are good and bad things about ports, at least mine. From what I understand they can be implanted many different ways. Mine was put in about one inch below my right collar bone, with a tube running up my neck. All my chemo treatments plus other medications have gone through my port. The port has held up beautifully and naturally my veins are in perfect shape. The annoying part is the tube up my neck. I can see and feel it all the time. If you were to look at my neck, it probably looks like a vein that sticks out a bit too much. But I see the tube. And there is the constant pressure in that area. I can feel it when I swallow, cough, talk, laugh, etc. Don't get me wrong, that annoyance is better then having screwed up veins forever, but it is irritating. You just get used to being annoyed. There's that word just again.

In addition to having the port put in, I also had to have a PET/CT scan and a MUGA scan. I had heard of a CT and PET scan, but I never heard of a MUGA scan before. MUGA stands for Multiple Gated Acquisition scan. It is the easiest and fastest of those 3 tests to take, and very important. The MUGA looks at all the facets of your working heart. When you do it before chemo, it gives the doctor a baseline of what your heart looks like now and how well it's pumping. After chemo is completed you do it again to see how much damage was done to it. Let's not kid ourselves here; when you're on a chemotherapy treatment, you're putting poison into your body on a regular bases, and lots of it. That poison is killing the cancer cells, but doesn't do the rest of your body much good. So it's very important to know, when it's over, if any severe damage was done to your heart that may need treatment.

All the scans came back fine. I make a point of asking if any cancer was spotted in my bones, luckily there isn't. Now it's a waiting game, June 4th is my first chemo treatment.

Ch. 8

CHEMO BEGINS

June 4th, a day that will live in infamy. Ok not really but a day I can't forget.

I get to the office right on time, and I have to say this is usually a good office. When an appointment is made they usually take you pretty much on time. How many doctors' offices can you say that about?

Anyway, the chemo is not actually administered by a doctor. There are doctors in the office in case there is a problem, but nurses do all the work. First thing that's done is a CBC (complete blood count). CBCs will become a regular thing for every chemo patient, and for most of us so will shots of some kind.

After my CBC I take a seat in the infusion room. This room is medium sized and can seat 6 people receiving treatment at one time. In addition, there are extra seats for people who bring a friend or a loved one with them. I brought Matt with me for my first trip. In subsequent sessions I came alone. It's a long and boring process and there really was no need for him to sit there for the whole time. It was a bit unnerving the first time, because on the day I went I was the youngest there by about 30 years. At first it felt strange, but then I realized I was glad that was true. That means that not that many "young" people had it. Unfortunately, in future sessions I saw many people under the age of 50.

The nurse, Diane, brought a bunch of bags to where I was sitting. She also had an unusually bent, big needle. She explained to me that this is the only kind of needle that should be used in this type of port. In case I have an emergency where I need to go to the ER, never let anyone attempt to use the port without this kind of needle. She hangs up the bags and cleans the area around my port, then prepares to put that big needle in me. "1-2-3 deep breath". Truth is, it really didn't hurt that much. When I saw that thing, I was expecting it to just kill. It's not just long and bent, but it's a thick needle. But since the port is just below the skin there really isn't that much tissue to go through. Little tissue, little pain I guess.

Now everyone is on a different kind of drug, and even people on the same drugs may be given them in different strengths and possibly different orders. So I can only speak about what I had and how it affected me.

First, I was given some premeds and hormones; honestly I couldn't even tell you what they were. The chemo drugs were Adriamycin and Cytoxin. Cytoxin took about 3 hours to administer. The Adriamycin takes about 10 minutes. It's put in what looks like a huge syringe, but without a needle. That syringe is attached to an IV tube and the liquid is "pushed" into me. The liquid is very red, fire engine red. And I was warned that my liquids will turn red for days to come. By the way, they aren't kidding about that. If you wear contact lenses you can stain them. When you urinate, you look like you're urinating blood. Don't be shocked. The more water you drink the quicker that will go away. But it still lasts for days.

After the treatment I felt fine. I was given a prescription for Ondansetron, which is supposed to combat nausea, and was told to drink lots and lots of water. I was fine for about 8 hours. Ondansetron is a pill, and I must say this is the most useless pill on the planet. To give a pill, any pill, to someone with extreme nausea is just plain stupid. For those of you who are doctors or nurses, lets see if I can make it clear to you. People that have trouble keeping down water cannot swallow pills.

Luckily, I have friends. And my family has friends. And my Temple is full of friends. One of these friends is named Myra. I think I've known her since I'm 5 years old, maybe before. She's just always been a part of my life. She is also one of the best pastry chefs you could ever hope to know. Here is a trick for those of you who may not have thought of it, like me. One thing that helps settle stomachs is ginger. I don't happen to like ginger ale, but I do like ginger snaps. Myra made me a huge 2 gallon bag full of the most delicious ginger snaps. Slowly I was able to swallow them, one nibble at a time, and with them water. Water is so important when you are going through chemo, the entire process dehydrates you. I don't mean your skin gets dry type of dehydration. I mean your eyes hurt from lack of moisture. It's that bad. Anyway, thanks Myra, you made those first few treatments bearable.

So several days pass, and I need to go in for a CBC (complete blood count). This is to check to make sure that not too many of my white or red blood cells have been destroyed in this process. So far so good. My count is fine and everything is progressing swimmingly. In fact when I get to the office I comment to Camille that I haven't lost any hair yet, which made me very happy. She just responded "just wait, because it will probably happen".

Well that didn't sound too good to me. I'd probably have no hair and couldn't afford a wig either. Back to Penny at Temple Beth Chai for more advice. She told me about the Walk for Beauty fund. I contacted them, filled out the paperwork and had my doctor sign a form, and made an appointment for a wig fitting. About 9 days later I had my wig, right in time for my hair to fall out. It was amazing and I can't thank them enough. Yes my hair did fall out, about 2 ½ weeks after my first chemo session it started. It didn't fall out in clumps; it was like it was thinning. You know when you run your fingers through your hair and you get a few stray hairs in your hand? That's what it was like except my hand was full. And no matter how many times I would run my fingers through my hair, it would always be full. Enough was enough.

When I got home from work one day, we decided to have a shaving party. We took my husband's beard trimmer and the kids helped me to shave it all off. It wasn't exactly a great job, but it did the trick. Also when it was gone I was able to see just how much hair I actually did lose. There were huge bald spots all over my head. It took about 5 minutes to get used to how I looked, and I promised myself that I wouldn't wear the wig around the house. I didn't want the kids to be scared. It's just that this was how mommy is now and hopefully mommy's hair will grow back soon.

Ch. 9

MY 15 MINUTES OF FAME

Back in March, while I was home recovering from the biopsy surgery, I saw Sen. John Edwards and his wife at a press conference. They wanted to announce that Elizabeth has breast cancer again, and that it spread into her bones.

At that time, I admit to feeling very selfish. After all, my world was crashing down on me. No money, no health insurance, 2 young kids, and awaiting biopsy results. So feeling sorry for Mrs. Edwards wasn't exactly top priority for me. Instead what I heard out of her press conference was this:

1) She thought she had a problem completely unrelated to cancer
2) After doing an x-ray, the doctor spotted something strange
3) They did more tests
4) They did a biopsy
5) They got the diagnosis from the biopsy
6) She began a new treatment
7) This entire series of events took about 48 hours

By the time this press conference took place, March 22nd, it was about a month from the time I found the lump to the time I had my biopsy, and hadn't had the official results yet. To say the least, I was jealous.

On June 23rd, I was watching CNN and saw a commercial for the upcoming Youtube / CNN debate. People could make videos and CNN might choose yours to show the candidates so they can answer them. Well, I was still jealous. I sent in a video. Anyone watching may not have realized it, but I was really talking to John Edwards. I wanted to know what he would do so that I could get the same kind of care his wife had.

As the debate got closer, my video started getting attention. To this day I don't really know why. People said it was stark, gripping, and moving. I guess the fact that I removed my wig just touched people. I started getting calls from newspapers and TV shows from all over the country. I got a call from one guy who was interested in creating a kind of "Extreme Makeover, Medical Addition". They even started calling me at work, which was annoying to say the least. I mean I'm working, leave me alone!

My video did make it into the debate, in a group of several health related videos. I don't think anyone really answered the question though. What I heard was Sen. Obama saying "I have a plan" and Sen. Edwards saying "I have a plan and its more inclusive then Sen. Obama's plan" and Sen. Clinton saying "I have a plan but that's not important, we need to change the outlook we have on health insurance first". No offense guys and gals, I want a plan. Deal with the outlook later. We need healthcare and we need it now.

After the debate and a very cool interview on CNN that I had a few days after that, my 15 min of fame was pretty much over. And I was glad. Not that it wasn't about the most exciting thing to probably happen in my life so far, and thank you Shira for inviting me to the program, but I think you have to be a certain kind of person to like that kind of attention, and it's not me. I did a video because I was mad and jealous. Some things did come out of it though.

A few people started offering me stuff like new wigs and trips to places for the kids that I can't afford. I was able to turn most of this stuff toward charities to help others. I also asked people who wanted to donate money someplace (but not to me) to give it to Planned Parenthood. Without their help I don't know where I would be.

Ch. 10

TREATMENT 2 WITH SHOTS

June 18th I go for another CBC, and this time my white blood cell count has plummeted, and I begin a Leukine regiment. I'm supposed to get shots daily for 5-7 days. So every day I head down to the office and get a shot during lunch time. By day 3 my bones start aching. By day 6 my back is just killing me. June 25th was my second treatment. I was feeling pretty good going into it aside from my back bothering me. We take a CBC first and the Leukine did the trick. My count was way up. Also I knew how to beat the nausea that would come without even having to take their pills, I defeated the hair thing, and I could even work through most of it. Luckily my eyebrows and eyelashes didn't fall out, so I didn't look too freakish. All in all, I was feeling pretty good.

I went alone this time, and found that it really wasn't a problem. I don't feel any effect from the drugs for about 8-12 hours after treatment, so that leaves plenty of time to go home and get sick. I fell asleep in the infusion room so time passed quickly. When I got home I was all ready for what would happen, I thought.

Tuesday morning I wake up, and I'm actually feeling decent. I'm tired, but ok. I can't seem to drink anything; I'm too nauseous for that. I can't even eat any ginger snaps. Oh well, I'm ok. I'm not even thirsty. I know the nurse told me to drink plenty of water, but no biggie. If I really needed it, I'd be thirsty. Right? I tried to take that stupid pill again, but I just can't swallow it. But I'm not hungry, not thirsty, and not worrying about it.

Wednesday rolls around, I'm still feeling surprisingly well. I'm tired, more tired then the day before, but ok. I call work and tell them that I might try to make it in for a few hours. But every time I try to get moving, I just can't. By 10am it's like every muscle in my body, even my brain went to sleep. All I can do is lie there. I'm still not hungry and not thirsty. I'm just tired. Tomorrow is another day. I call my office with the news that I'll try again tomorrow.

Thursday I'm scheduled to have a CBC, so I have to get up and get to that. I hadn't made any arrangements for anyone to take me, because of how I felt last time, so I just must go myself. It takes me until about noon to actually get up out of bed without literally falling back into it. But I do it. I put on my work clothes just in case I manage to make it in. I drive the half hour to my doctor's office for my CBC. My numbers are good. Not great, but good enough. I'll have to come back next week for another CBC to make sure the numbers stay high enough.

I walk out of his office thinking "hey I'm still walking". If I can do this, I'm sure I can work a little. Even just a couple of hours. After all, it's not like I get paid for time off. Every hour I take off is an hour I'm not getting paid. And I need the money badly. My doctor's office isn't far from work, so I head over there. When get to work I park in my spot, I just sit looking at the door for a minute. I want to go in, but I just can't move. I decide to put on the radio, open the window and just rest in my car for a few minutes. Forty-five minutes later my strength seemed to have returned a little, so I head inside.

I walk into the office and everyone is surprised to see me. They are all looking at me in a very concerned way though. I didn't know it at the time, but I was pasty white. I told everyone I was fine and asked to clock in. Here is what I'm told happened next. I go to my supervisor's, Diana's, desk. I clock in, sit down and pass out. That's how quick it was. I'm not sure how long I was out really, just a few seconds to a couple of minutes I'd guess. When I came too, it felt like half the office was standing over me. The manager asked who she could get to help me, because there was no way they were letting me drive out of there. Should they call 911 or call my husband, what? I knew Matt was home with our little one and Mom was actually much closer. I had them call her to bring me back to the doctor's office. He was on the same property as a hospital, just in case we needed that.

Well naturally you can guess what happened. My body was completely dehydrated. For the next few hours they pumped me full of liquids through my port. I was feeling much better when they were done. I told them I couldn't swallow the pills they gave me. I tried and tried, but can't do it. Finally they gave me something useful. There is a product Ondansetron ODT (orally dissolving tablets). Same drug, but now it's in a tablet that dissolves in your mouth in 5 seconds. Well THIS I can take! It's not quite as strong as the pills apparently, but between those and the ginger snaps, now I can make it through the rest of this. I actually needed another infusion on Saturday, but not for as long, just kind of "topping off" my tank, if you will.

While I was there they did a CBC on me instead of waiting until Monday. Sure enough my white blood cell count was already down. By the way, this is known as leucopenia. A normal count should be between 4,300 and 10,800 cells per cubic millimeter (cmm). In order to be allowed to take my next treatment, I have to have at least 1,500 per cmm. Mine has dropped to about 1,000. Time for more drugs. I'm going to be given daily shots of Leukine again. This is supposed to activate my bone marrow and get it to produce more white blood cells. It's mostly used for leukemia and bone marrow transfer patients. So a 7 day treatment is ordered.

Now I know for a fact that my reactions to Leukine are my own and not everyone has them. I would sit and talk with other people in the infusion rooms at my doctors offices (he has 2). Many of these people had no real reaction to the Leukine except for the increased white blood cell production. That just was not the case for me.

Ch. 11

THE SHOTS CONTINUE

I begin my Leukine regimen on June 28th. I have appointments set for 7 days of shots, with 2 CBCs during that time. My oncologist's offices are open Saturday and Sunday for a few hours so people can get their needed medicine.

On day 5, Monday, I have a CBC again and my count has dropped even more, its down near 800 now. So they want me to keep taking shots and, on Friday, I'll have another CBC. That would be 9 shots in a row, but I'm told that I need it. Friday comes and my count is back up to 1000, but that's still not high enough. We decide I should take the weekend off from shots, perhaps my bone marrow is working and it's just not showing in the tests yet. I have another CBC Monday, and it's STILL around 1000. They decide to give me more shots. Thursday I go for a CBC yet again, I'm up to about 1300, that's close but not good enough. Mind you now, I've had 13 shots in 15 days. The nurses tell me that there is better and stronger medication, but that Medicaid won't pay for it unless I have no choice but to use it for some reason. I was about to reach the point of "no choice".

Friday, July 13, I go to the office once more and get my 14th shot. I get about 10 minutes from the office, maybe less, and I can't see. I'm driving on what is a pretty major road and all of a sudden all the blood rushed to my head. I couldn't think, couldn't see anything, and got incredibly hot. If I had my wits about me at all, I would have pulled over, but I didn't. Somehow, I made it home alive. My husband took me straight to the emergency room, because something was very wrong.

I'm not sure how long I was there, I think about 6 hours. From what I understand, I became allergic to Leukine. I have no allergies to anything, so it was quite a shock to me to have this result. It's not unheard of though. They hydrated me, gave me Benadryl, and when I was strong enough they sent me home.   On Saturday, I went to the doctor's office again and told them they had to find something else, because I wasn't going to take the Leukine. They said that my white blood cell count should be high enough on Monday for my next treatment, and they would figure out my next step by then.

Now I can't reiterate enough, this was my reaction and my reaction alone. When I sit in the office talking to the other patients, many of them are on Leukine and have been for months. They do not have allergic reactions and after 5 days or so, their white blood cell count rebounds with no problems. So yes in this case it was one of those "everyone is different" situations.

July 16th is treatment 3 for me, that goes pretty well and with the new ODT medication and ginger snaps I can drink plenty of water. I can't really eat anything for 5 days besides the snaps, but that's not important. The water is what's important and I have no trouble keeping that down. Water really is the key to this whole thing.

July 23rd I go for a CBC and my count once again is down around the 1000 mark. Shots again. This time we switch to Neupogen. It's a 3-5 day regimen, normally. We test me again after 5 days of shots, and it seems to have worked. Thank goodness. I'm getting really tired of shots. Neupogen is stronger then Leukine so you take fewer shots overall, but also gave me stronger bone aches. There are times I would cry from the pain of it. But hey, just 5 more chemo treatments to go!

Ch. 12

MY KIDS AND GUILT

My kids are seven and three at the time I'm writing this book. As I've mentioned previously that my elder daughter has PDD, Pervasive Development Disorder; it's on the Autism spectrum. My younger daughter is "typically developing", aka normal.

I've tried to keep them from knowing too much, but there is no way you can keep everything away from them. Of course, losing my hair was the first and most pronounced thing they saw that was wrong. Being sick in bed for days was the next. At first we tried to keep them away as much as we could during those times. They would sleep over at Grandma's house a lot. But eventually that had to stop.

My eldest, Niki, doesn't really understand and can't express herself to well. Ironically, that makes her easier to deal with. I tell her I'm going to be OK and she accepts it. She was always Daddy's girl anyway, so he can distract her pretty easily when it's needed. She doesn't really ask questions unless I'm in the hospital. My youngest is much harder.

Samantha is inquisitive, intuitive, vocal, verbal, empathic, and sometimes a royal pain in the tush. But that last part comes with being 3. She's truly Mommy's girl and has been since birth.

She likes to "snuggle" with me. After my first treatment when I got sick, she got really scared and was afraid to touch me. She knew where my port was, because she had seen the bandage on my chest. I had to gently show her that she could touch me. Even now we still struggle a bit. A few days ago (as I'm writing this) out of the clear blue she said "I'll always remember you Mommy". It took every ounce in my body not to cry at that. Almost daily they ask if I'm getting healthy yet. I tell them that I'm getting healthier every day and even though the medicine I'm taking makes me sick sometimes, by next summer I'll be healthy and strong and we'll be able to go to the beach. Something I couldn't do once this year.

The irony is, when they started asking these questions was when I stopped having my nightmares. The more I wanted to reassure them, the more I had to convince myself that what I was saying was true. I'm not a good liar. So since I determined that, while I may not tell them everything, I would not lie to my kids, I had to believe what I was saying. The more I answered their questions, the better I felt. You see I often come home with bandages on my arms from the shots of Leukine and then Neupogen (they have to be shot into fatty tissue subcutaneously so they can't be put in my port). Eventually I would take them with me when they didn't have school. After all, if I could see them get their vaccinations and tell them the whole time that this was good for them and would only hurt for a second, they should be able to see me get a shot, right?

It did work though, and even today when one of them asks "are you getting healthy Mommy" I can look them straight in the eye and say "Yes I am". I gained a new understand of life. I used to hear people say that they were able to get through a difficult situation because of their kids. I didn't understand it until now.

Ch. 13

HAPPY BIRTHDAY TO ME

I just had my 36th birthday. I've never been a person who looks forward to or tries to hide from my birthday. It just doesn't matter that much to me. But as this year's birthday is passing, I do something unusual. I reflect on what has happened. My first 35 years seemed so uneventful, normal, etc. This year, everything is going wrong. From hitting rock bottom financially to breast cancer, which makes money problems seem like nothing. Yet what has happened has made me appreciate those around me so much more.

My kids, well I talked about them in the last chapter. My husband, who by this point has finally gotten a full time job, has shown me a new tenderness that I don't know if even he knew he was capable of. My family (parents, aunts, uncles, grandparents), have always been close, but now it seems that not a week goes by where at least one of them isn't helping with something. My best friends; Ivy can always make me laugh no matter how hard I'm crying and Paulette has been with me through thick, thin, and worst of all…. high school! My in-laws have made trips here whenever they could and called regularly. Temple Beth Chai of Hauppauge, the members of who have helped me with the best advice, cookies, and even some money on occasion. Suffolk Federal Credit Union, my fellow employees have done so much for me. I have to give a special shout out to Rena, Diana, Nini, James, Melissa, Briana, Jess, and everyone that I've worked with. Without their help and understanding, well I don't know if I could have asked to be with a better group of people.

And last, but by no means least, is my Mom, who should have her own place in the "Most incredible Mom" hall of fame. I would have to add 5 pages to this book to describe all she has done to help me. I know some people say that their mothers are always there when they need them, but mine proves it everyday. She drives 2 hours round trip 5 days a week to get Niki off the school bus. She watches Samantha 3 days a week (sometimes more). She takes care of them every vacation. She drives me around when I'm too sick to drive myself. She comes to my house to watch over me on days my chemo is especially bad. Heck she even helped my husband find his job! There is no way I could go into everything in enough detail to describe all she has done for me, and continues to do. She is one of a kind.

Next year I hope to actually celebrate my birthday. Nothing fancy, just a nice cake. For me that actually is a celebration! I think from now on I'll commemorate every year that passes, because for a while I was afraid that I may not have anymore.

Ch. 14

TREATMENTS FOUR AND FIVE

I wish I could say that by now I've gotten into a routine with the treatments, but truth is that every one is different. My body's reaction is different with every treatment.

This is my last treatment with the Cytoxin / Adriamycin combination. I feel very weak after this treatment. It seems to have hit me a bit faster. Once again, nausea doesn't seem to be a big problem this time, but I sleep for days. Oh well, when your body tells you that you need to sleep its best to listen to it.

One thing I'd like to mention at this point is hair loss. When people think of chemo and hair loss, they think about the head. Also they tend to think that it all comes out at once, at least that's what I thought would happen. Not so.

After I shaved my head, I noticed slowly that all the stubble started disappearing. It took weeks. I don't think it was until my 4th treatment that it stopped, leaving a little bit around my ears and nape of my neck. The rest was gone. My eyebrows and eyelashes at this point were still intact. But what people don't tell you about is losing the rest of your hair. If you think of a place you have hair, you can lose it, in whole or in part. My underarm hair, gone. Leg hair, gone. Well ok those were two good things. It also feels like I got a Brazilian wax, which is pretty cool. But the hard one to deal with for me was losing my nose hair. It didn't all go at any point, but its constant slow trickle of falling out made it so I was constantly sneezing.

After treatment 4 I made an appointment for my Neupogen shots. At this point we knew that it's simply a fact of my chemo that my white blood cell count is going to drop. There is another medication on the market called Neulasta. The advantage of this medication is that you take only one shot instead of a series of shots. After the YouTube Democratic debate Senator Clinton's office called me to see if they could help me with anything. I explained that certain medications are not covered by Medicaid. Her office worked on this problem and I am proud to say that it is now being covered by New York Medicaid. Unfortunately, I was no longer on Medicaid. I now had insurance through my job and they won't pay for it! Oh well. Back to daily shots.

They seem to be much harder on me this time. I'm not kidding you when I say that at times I would lay bed crying from the pain in my bones. A few times it would hit me while I was at work, and I wouldn't be able to bend over to do things. This hurts many bones at the same time, than moves to another location. So for a while my back and neck would hurt, then it would move to my arms or legs. It would be difficult to stay still and yet it was difficult to move.

August 27th was my first treatment on my new chemo drug. This drug is called Taxotere. It seems that each drug can affect cancer in different ways, so the first set did all it could do and now this one will do what it does.

As I was given the chemo, I started to feel a tightening in my chest. My nurses and the doctor immediately jump to action. I was given something called Dexamethasone in my IV before restarting the Taxotere. For my next treatment I will be given a prescription of Dexamethasone to take for three days. I should take it the day before, the day of, and after my treatment as a precautionary measure.

Just as with the previous chemo drugs, my white blood cell count dropped with the new ones. Also my eyebrows and eyelashes immediately fell out. It looks very strange, and I'm not someone who wears makeup generally at all. So when I try to put on eye brow pencil it looks like clown makeup. I really wish I could get the TV makeup guys from CNN to do it for me!

Ch. 15

MY BIG MISTAKE

It's amazing how fast everything seems to be going now. Unlike the other chemo drugs, the Taxotere doesn't make me nauseous. This is such an incredible relief to me that I've been eating everything under the sun. My white blood cell count still drops, so I still have to have those painful shots… but I can eat! The best diet I've ever been on in my life is Chemo, I've lost 25 lbs. But now I'll eat a lot of that back. Oh well.

September 17 comes, and it's time for treatment 6. One problem, I forgot all about the Dexamethasone. When I get to the office they ask me if I took it and I sheepishly said no. They gave me an IV of it, and then started the Taxotere. BIG MISTAKE. It only took a couple of seconds for my chest to freeze up to the point where I could hardly breathe. The nurses immediately stopped the treatment of course.

Remember, all these drugs are cumulative. Each one affects you harder then the previous dose. So this one hit me much harder and faster then the last one. They hooked me up to an oxygen tank for a while until the symptoms passed. Well I sure learned my lesson that time! We rescheduled for Thursday and I swore I'd never miss taking needed medicine again. The last thing I want to do is drag out this process longer then I have to.

Wednesday and Thursday morning I take my Dexamethasone and Thursday afternoon we reattempt treatment, this time with no problems.

So here is the next lesson my friends. While often the doctors and nurses don't tell you enough, when they do tell you to do something… do it!

Ch. 16

NEARING THE END

These treatments went as well as my second attempt at number 6. I was feeling much better with the Taxotere treatments. I didn't have to take as much time off of work, although my white blood cell count did drop and I still had to go for daily Neupogen.

By this point I dreaded 2 things more then anything, first off those damn shots. The pain in my bones doesn't seem to go away at any point in between treatments. I know it means the medicine is working, building up my white blood cells. But being in constant pain and not getting a lot of sleep is hard. I would take Tylenol or other pain relievers but they never helped that much.

Secondly, I had developed what is affectionately known as "chemo brain". At times I seemed to have no short term memory. It's very disconcerting. I had begun to write things down and leave notes all over the place, otherwise I'd forget everything. Even so, many things just slipped. At work, if someone asked me to do something I would have to do it that very second. I became afraid if I didn't, I wouldn't remember to do it later. Even 10 minutes was too long to wait.

As I write this, it's been 2 months since my final chemo treatment, and my brain still doesn't seem to be up to speed.

But on the whole, I was ok. My last treatment was November 1st. Everyone at work was so happy for me that we actually had a little party. It's nice to have your coworkers pulling for you. So here I was, feeling I was over the worst of it. Then I got a cold.

Ch. 17

WHEN IS A COLD NOT A COLD?

The answer to that question is when it happens during chemo. If your temperature goes above 100.5 degrees, you're supposed to tell your doctor immediately

I developed a cold, just one of those annoying fall/winter colds that I usually get every year at some point. I checked my temperature before going to work and didn't have one, so I didn't worry. I was coughing up yellow gunk, but no fever.

During work I did what I had been doing all these many months. I planned to take an extended lunch so I would have time to get to the doctor's office for my shot. But when I got there and my nose was running and I was coughing to the point where my chest really hurt, the nurses went into full alert mode.

They took my temperature and it was over 101 degrees. Now I wasn't allowed to leave. They immediately had me admitted to the nearby hospital. I called work over and over, because it went from the idea that I was going in to be looked over to the idea that I was going to be overnight to the fact that I ended up being there almost a week.

I was given so many antibiotics via IV that I lost track of them all. They were never actually able to figure out what I had. At one point, they thought my port had gotten infected. This apparently is not an uncommon occurrence. Neither is going into the hospital for a cold. When you have no white blood cells, having a cold could be extremely dangerous.

I was put on what is called a neutropenic diet. Basically the idea is to keep your food as clean and free of germs as humanly possible. So I could have no rare meat, which is my preference. Also no raw vegetables or fruits, no sliced cheeses or meats, no tap or spring water (it must be distilled), and most interestingly of all, no pepper. Apparently pepper is a very dirty condiment, so unless it was cooked into the food I couldn't have it at all. Even then, they would prefer I not have it at all, just in case.

So there I was for 6 days, on 24 hour infusion of water and varying antibiotics... and bored to tears. After 3 days I stopped coughing and my fever went away. My cold stopped after 5 days, but I wasn't allowed to leave until they figured out what was causing my sickness or until I cried unmercifully wanting to go home. The crying came first.

Their infection specialist was never able to figure out what it was that made me sick. I still say it was just a cold. It was just made all the worse because of the whole lack of white blood cell count thing. But better safe then sorry. Yes I missed my family and lost a lot of money being out of work. But a simple cold could lead to death if you don't have the resources to fight it. That's a pretty scary thought, dying from a cold.

Ch. 18

MY STORY ENDS WITH A BANG

At this point I'm done with chemo and will be going in for surgery to remove what is left of my lump soon. Then I'll have radiation. But first I got a big shock.

I went for a follow up Pet/Ct scan to see if there were any traces of cancer remaining. After the results came back, I had a consultation with my oncologist. He showed me the results of the first scan and the follow up.

As you may recall, after the first scan I didn't see the results. I just asked if it was in my bones. Well as it turns out, the cancer was much worse then I knew. I had a second lump under the first and it was in lymph nodes in the middle of my chest and under my arm. So it had already started spreading.

If I hadn't found it and gotten treatment quickly, well now almost a year later I could be on my deathbed instead of knowing that I'll be able to watch my girls grow up. That's a tremendous difference.

I'm happy to say that my follow up scan shows no traces of cancer. Ultimately I think it was better for me not to know how bad it was early on. It probably would have made things much harder, knowing how bad it really was. It might have affected how my body responded to the treatment, and it might not have responded as well as it did. At this point what is left of the lump is so small you can't even feel it. I'm looking forward to it being removed though.

In fact, a follow up MRI showed that the smaller lump has disappeared completely and the big lump is now a mere 17mm by 5mm. The treatment worked beyond what I could have imagined. My breast will definitely be saved now.

This is where my story ends, at least for now. Just knowing I will live, which is good enough for me.

Ch. 19

What I've learned

There is so much people can learn about themselves from being sick. Being in bed for days at a time, and yet trying to go on with life, leaves you with a lot of time to think.

First of all, I learned how weak I can be. I had never been a person to cry over things unless someone died. Yet at the beginning I would cry all the time. But I believe it was cathartic. I needed to do it in order to move on, to perhaps mourn the death of the old me and bring on a stronger one.

Secondly, I learned that no doctor no matter how qualified; is the be all and end all of information and knowledge. The first surgeon I saw wanted to do a double mastectomy on me. The second did too, plus his surgery caused me to have a raging infection. The third has saved my breasts and my life. As wonderful as he is, he couldn't do everything for me. I'd read about medications and treatment on my own, both to back up what he was saying and because he wouldn't tell me everything. Knowledge is important for a patient, and must never be taken for granted.

Thirdly, life must go on. Unless you are lucky enough to be rich enough to not need your salary, you must work through this process. If you are lucky enough to not need a salary, I'd recommend doing volunteer work. Having something to do when you're not sick is very important. It brings your life into focus and reminds you that your illness is only one facet of what is happening in your life, not your entire life.

Lastly, get involved politically. As I said at the beginning, I wanted to be a Senator. Someday, who knows, maybe I will be. But I'll tell you one thing, I'm not going away. For issues I believe in, like universal healthcare and energy independence, I intend on being a thorn in every politician's side I can. I call and email my Senator's and Congressman's offices regularly. I firmly believe that my moment in the CNN / Youtube debate is something that has kept healthcare in the headlines all these months later. I will not allow that issue to die as long as I have breath in my body.

And thanks to this treatment, I will have that breath for a very, very long time.

SPECIAL THANKS

I can't end this book without a bunch of thank you's to everyone.

First off, once again to my Mom, she has made my life bearable.

Secondly to the rest of my family for always being there for me, I love you all.

Thirdly to my two best friends Ivy and Paulette. We can't talk everyday, but you're both in my thoughts constantly. I don't know what I'd do without you two in my life.

And finally to:

Temple Beth Chai – Especially (in alphabetical order) Beverly, Fran, Gina, Myra, Penny, and the Rabbi.

Suffolk Federal Credit Union – for giving me a new home.

KWS/OMWF/Whatever the name of the guild is now – your love and support has meant so much to me.

The gang at RRMB – thanks for both your caring about a stranger and helping me take my mind off things.

CNN – for helping get the message of national healthcare on the front pages.

Diane and Camille at the Oncologist's office – they made sitting there for hours on end bearable and at times even fun.

www.ingramcontent.com/pod-product-compliance
Lightning Source LLC
Chambersburg PA
CBHW022133280326
41933CB00007B/675